LOW FAT DOG FOOD FOR PANCREATITIS

Nutrient-Packed Canine Cuisine: Low-Fat Dog Food
Ideal for Pancreatitis Support

Dr. Melissa R. Steven

INTRODUCTION

Welcome to "Low Fat Dog Food for Pancreatitis," a comprehensive guide crafted with the utmost care and expertise to illuminate the path toward optimal health for your canine confidant. Pancreatitis, a condition characterized by inflammation of the pancreas, demands a nuanced approach to dietary management. As we embark on this journey together, we will delve into the intricate interplay of nutrition and well-being, navigating the maze of low-fat diets tailored to alleviate the burdens of pancreatitis.

This guide is more than a compendium of instructions; it is a beacon of knowledge, providing insights into the intricacies of canine nutrition and offering practical solutions to empower you as the primary steward of your dog's health. Our journey encompasses the realms of commercial low-fat dog foods, carefully curated homemade recipes, and the delicate art of introducing new foods. We will unravel the enigma of supplements, explore feeding strategies, and address the common pitfalls that may lurk along the path to recovery.

Beyond the realms of practical advice, this guide endeavors to inspire through the sharing of success stories and the resilience displayed by our canine counterparts. In the pursuit of a healthier, happier existence for your furry friend, we invite you to embark on a transformative odyssey—one that transcends the realm of mere sustenance to embrace the profound connection between nutrition and vitality.

As we venture forth, let this guide be your compass, guiding you through the labyrinth of low-fat dietary choices with a blend of scientific understanding and compassionate care. May the pages that follow be a source of enlightenment, a roadmap to a healthier, more vibrant life for your cherished companion. Together, let us embark on a journey toward canine wellness, where each bite becomes a step toward renewed vigor, and each chapter unfolds a narrative of resilience, love, and the unwavering bond between human and hound.

TABLE OF CONTENTS

1.1 Understanding Pancreatitis in Dogs

Pancreatitis, a term that echoes with concern for dog owners, is a condition characterized by inflammation of the pancreas—an organ crucial for digestion and metabolic regulation. To comprehend the impact of pancreatitis on our canine companions, it is essential to unravel the intricacies of this physiological disruption.

1. The Pancreatic Role:
The pancreas, nestled near the stomach, plays a pivotal role in digestion by secreting enzymes responsible for breaking down fats, proteins, and carbohydrates. Additionally, it produces insulin, a key player in regulating blood sugar levels. When inflammation occurs, this harmonious process is disrupted.

2. Causes of Pancreatitis:
Pancreatitis in dogs can be triggered by various factors. Dietary indiscretions, such as consuming high-fat foods or scavenging from the trash, are common culprits. Other potential causes include obesity, certain medications, genetics, and underlying health conditions.

3. Clinical Signs:

Recognizing the signs of pancreatitis is crucial for early intervention. Symptoms may range from mild gastrointestinal distress, such as vomiting and diarrhea, to more severe indications like abdominal pain, lethargy, and a reluctance to eat. It's essential to note that these signs can mimic other health issues, underscoring the importance of veterinary evaluation.

4. Diagnosing Pancreatitis:

Accurate diagnosis often involves a combination of clinical symptoms, blood tests measuring pancreatic enzymes, and imaging studies like ultrasound. Your veterinarian will employ a comprehensive approach to confirm the presence and severity of pancreatitis.

5. Acute vs. Chronic Pancreatitis:

Pancreatitis is categorized into acute and chronic forms. Acute cases typically manifest suddenly and can be severe, requiring immediate attention. Chronic pancreatitis, on the other hand, involves prolonged inflammation, often leading to gradual and recurring symptoms.

6. Treatment and Management:
The treatment plan for pancreatitis aims to alleviate symptoms, restore digestive balance, and address underlying causes. This may involve a period of fasting, intravenous fluids, and a low-fat diet tailored to ease the strain on the pancreas.

7. Prevention Strategies:
While certain factors leading to pancreatitis may be unavoidable, preventive measures include maintaining a balanced, low-fat diet, avoiding feeding table scraps, and ensuring your dog's weight remains within a healthy range. Regular veterinary check-ups contribute to early detection and intervention.

Understanding pancreatitis is the cornerstone of proactive canine care. By recognizing the signs, seeking prompt veterinary attention, and implementing preventive measures, dog owners can play a pivotal role in safeguarding the digestive health of their cherished companions.

1.2 Importance of Low-Fat Diets

A dog's well-being is intricately linked to its diet, and when it comes to certain health conditions, such as pancreatitis, the role of nutrition becomes paramount. Understanding the importance of low-fat diets for dogs goes beyond culinary choices; it becomes a cornerstone in managing and preventing various health issues.

1. Pancreatitis Management:
One of the primary reasons for adopting a low-fat diet for dogs is the management of pancreatitis. Dogs diagnosed with pancreatitis often struggle to process and metabolize dietary fats. By reducing the fat content in their meals, the workload on the pancreas is lessened, promoting a smoother digestive process and mitigating the risk of inflammation.

2. Digestive Health:
Low-fat diets contribute to overall digestive health in dogs. Excessive dietary fat can lead to gastrointestinal upset, causing symptoms like vomiting, diarrhea, and abdominal discomfort. Opting for a diet with moderate fat levels supports a gentler digestion process, reducing the likelihood of digestive disturbances.

3. Weight Management:

Keeping a solid weight is critical for a canine's general wellbeing and life span. Low-fat diets aid in weight management, preventing obesity—an established risk factor for pancreatitis and various other health issues. By promoting lean body mass and controlling calorie intake, these diets contribute to an ideal body condition.

4. Cardiovascular Health:

High-fat diets can contribute to the development of cardiovascular issues in dogs. By adopting a low-fat approach, pet owners can help safeguard their canine companions against conditions such as heart disease and hypertension. This nutritional strategy supports not only digestive health but also the cardiovascular system.

5. Prevention of Gallbladder Issues:

Dogs on diets rich in fat may be at a higher risk of developing gallbladder problems. Low-fat diets can help prevent the formation of gallstones and reduce the strain on the gallbladder, contributing to a healthier and more balanced digestive system.

6. Joint and Mobility Support:
Certain low-fat diets are enriched with nutrients like omega-3 fatty acids, which play a role in joint health. By incorporating these essential nutrients, low-fat diets can contribute to improved joint function and mobility, particularly beneficial for older dogs or those prone to arthritis.

7. Long-Term Wellness:
Beyond immediate health concerns, the adoption of a low-fat diet sets the stage for long-term wellness. Preventing obesity, managing digestive issues, and supporting overall health lay the foundation for a fulfilling and active life for your furry friend.

The importance of low-fat diets for dogs extends beyond a mere dietary choice—it becomes a proactive step towards promoting health, preventing ailments, and nurturing a vibrant and joyful life for our canine companions. As conscientious caretakers, the nutritional decisions we make play a vital role in ensuring our dogs lead lives filled with vitality and well-being.

Dietary Guidelines for Pancreatitis

2.1 Nutritional Requirements for Dogs with Pancreatitis

Managing the nutritional needs of dogs diagnosed with pancreatitis demands a careful and tailored approach. The digestive challenges associated with this condition necessitate a focus on specific nutritional requirements to support overall health, aid in recovery, and prevent the recurrence of pancreatitis episodes.

1. Low-Fat Content:
The cornerstone of a diet for dogs with pancreatitis is a reduced fat content. Excessive dietary fats can trigger inflammation of the pancreas, exacerbating the condition. Opting for a low-fat diet lightens the digestive load, easing the strain on the pancreas and promoting a smoother digestion process.

2. Moderate Protein Levels:
While protein is a crucial component of a dog's diet, it's essential to maintain a balance. Dogs with pancreatitis may benefit from moderate protein levels to support muscle maintenance and overall health.

Lean protein sources, such as chicken or turkey, can be included while avoiding high-fat meats.

3. Complex Carbohydrates:
Incorporating complex carbohydrates is vital for providing a steady source of energy without overburdening the digestive system. Options like brown rice, sweet potatoes, and oatmeal can contribute to a well-rounded and easily digestible diet.

4. Digestible Fiber:
Including digestible fiber in the diet aids in promoting gastrointestinal health. Fiber helps regulate bowel movements and can be sourced from vegetables like pumpkin or carrots. However, excessive fiber should be avoided, as it may contribute to flatulence or other digestive issues.

5. Omega-3 Fatty Acids:
Omega-3 fatty acids, found in sources like fish oil, can have anti-inflammatory properties and support overall health. These essential fatty acids contribute to coat and skin health while potentially mitigating inflammation associated with pancreatitis.

6. Vitamins and Minerals:
Ensuring adequate levels of essential vitamins and minerals is crucial for dogs with pancreatitis. Supplements or foods rich in B vitamins, vitamin E, and zinc can contribute to overall well-being. However, it's important to consult with a veterinarian to determine specific supplementation needs.

7. Hydration:
Adequate hydration is paramount, especially during episodes of pancreatitis. Dogs may be prone to dehydration due to vomiting and decreased appetite. Wet or moistened food can contribute to overall fluid intake, and access to fresh water should be readily available.

8. Feeding Frequency and Portion Control:
Rather than large, infrequent meals, dividing daily food intake into smaller, more frequent portions can be beneficial. This approach helps manage digestion, reduces the workload on the pancreas, and minimizes the risk of triggering pancreatic inflammation.

9. Veterinary Guidance:
Every dog's nutritional needs are unique, and consulting with a veterinarian is imperative when

formulating a diet for a dog with pancreatitis. A veterinarian can assess the specific health conditions, tailor dietary recommendations, and monitor the dog's response to the prescribed nutrition plan.

Adhering to these nutritional guidelines provides a foundation for managing pancreatitis in dogs. Tailoring the diet to individual needs, monitoring for any adverse reactions, and collaborating closely with a veterinarian contribute to the well-being and long-term health of dogs grappling with pancreatitis.

2.2 Role of Low-Fat Dog Food in Managing Pancreatitis

Managing pancreatitis in dogs requires a vigilant and strategic approach, and the selection of an appropriate diet plays a pivotal role in mitigating the impact of this inflammatory condition. Low-fat dog food emerges as a crucial ally in this management strategy, addressing the specific needs of dogs grappling with pancreatitis.

1. Reducing Pancreatic Strain:
The primary objective of incorporating low-fat dog food is to alleviate the strain on the pancreas. Dogs with pancreatitis struggle to process and metabolize fats effectively, and a low-fat diet helps in moderating the workload on this vital digestive organ. By minimizing the fat content, the risk of exacerbating inflammation is diminished.

2. Preventing Pancreatic Stimulation:
High-fat meals can trigger the release of digestive enzymes from the pancreas, potentially leading to further inflammation. Low-fat dog food aims to provide essential nutrients without overstimulating the

pancreas, allowing for a controlled and less reactive digestive process.

3. Digestive Health Support:
Low-fat dog food is crafted to support optimal digestive health. With carefully selected ingredients that are easily digestible, these diets help minimize the risk of gastrointestinal upset. This is particularly crucial for dogs with pancreatitis, as they may be more prone to digestive disturbances.

4. Weight Management:
Obesity is a known risk factor for pancreatitis, and low-fat dog food contributes to weight management. By controlling the calorie content and promoting lean protein sources, these diets help maintain a healthy weight, reducing the likelihood of recurring pancreatitis episodes.

5. Balancing Essential Nutrients:
While reducing fat content is key, it's equally important to ensure that other essential nutrients are balanced in the diet. Low-fat dog food formulations aim to provide adequate levels of protein, carbohydrates, vitamins, and minerals to support

overall health without compromising nutritional requirements.

6. Transitioning to Home-Cooked Meals:
In some cases, pet owners may opt for home-cooked meals as part of a low-fat diet. These meals can be tailored to the specific needs of the dog, incorporating lean protein sources, complex carbohydrates, and minimal fats. However, it's crucial to work closely with a veterinarian to ensure a well-balanced and nutritionally complete diet.

7. Consistency and Long-Term Management:
Consistency is key in managing pancreatitis, and incorporating low-fat dog food as a long-term dietary strategy contributes to ongoing health maintenance. Regular monitoring, adjustments to the diet as needed, and collaboration with a veterinarian form a comprehensive approach to the sustained well-being of dogs with pancreatitis.

The role of low-fat dog food in managing pancreatitis extends beyond mere dietary restrictions. It embodies a tailored, holistic strategy aimed at supporting digestive health, preventing inflammation, and providing the essential nutrients dogs need for overall well-being. As a cornerstone in the management of pancreatitis, low-fat dog food becomes a proactive and nurturing choice, ensuring a balanced and fulfilling life for our canine companions.

2.3 Balancing Essential Nutrients

Ensuring that our canine companions receive a well-balanced diet is fundamental to their overall health, vitality, and longevity. Each nutrient serves a specific purpose in supporting various bodily functions, and achieving the right balance is crucial for promoting optimal well-being in dogs.

1. Protein:
Protein is a cornerstone of a dog's diet, playing a vital role in building and repairing tissues, maintaining muscle mass, and supporting immune function. High-quality protein sources, such as lean meats, fish, and eggs, contribute to the essential amino acids required for a dog's overall health.

2. Carbohydrates:
Carbohydrates serve as a primary energy source for dogs. While they are not strictly essential, incorporating complex carbohydrates like brown rice, sweet potatoes, and whole grains provides sustained energy, aids in digestion, and contributes to overall dietary balance.

3. Fats:

Fats are crucial for dogs as they provide a concentrated source of energy, support nutrient absorption, and contribute to coat and skin health. However, balancing fat intake is essential, especially for dogs with conditions like pancreatitis. Opting for healthy fats, such as those from fish oil or flaxseed, helps strike the right balance.

4. Vitamins:

Essential vitamins, including A, B complex, C, D, and E, play diverse roles in a dog's health. From supporting vision and immune function to promoting skin health and bone development, ensuring an adequate supply of vitamins is vital. A well-balanced diet usually provides these nutrients, but supplements may be necessary in specific cases.

5. Minerals:

Minerals like calcium, phosphorus, potassium, and zinc are crucial for bone health, nerve function, and overall physiological balance. A balanced diet with varied ingredients typically meets a dog's mineral requirements. However, care should be taken to avoid excesses or deficiencies.

6. Water:
Often overlooked but of paramount importance, water is a vital nutrient for dogs. It aids in digestion, regulates body temperature, and supports various bodily functions. Providing access to clean and fresh water is essential to maintain hydration and overall health.

7. Fiber:
Fiber is essential for digestive health, promoting regular bowel movements and preventing constipation. While not considered a primary nutrient, incorporating fiber from sources like vegetables and fruits supports gastrointestinal function and contributes to a balanced diet.

8. Omega-3 Fatty Acids:
Omega-3 fatty acids, found in fish oil, flaxseed, and certain fish varieties, offer anti-inflammatory properties. They contribute to skin and coat health, support joint function, and may have positive effects on cardiovascular health. Including these essential fatty acids helps achieve a well-rounded nutrient profile.

9. Antioxidants:
Antioxidants, found in fruits and vegetables, play a role in neutralizing free radicals and supporting immune

function. Including a variety of colorful, antioxidant-rich foods in a dog's diet helps promote overall health and may contribute to disease prevention.

10. Consulting with a Veterinarian:
Every dog is unique, and their nutritional needs may vary based on factors such as breed, age, health status, and activity level. Consulting with a veterinarian is crucial to tailor a diet that meets the specific requirements of an individual dog and ensures optimal health.

Balancing essential nutrients for dogs is an art that involves selecting high-quality ingredients, understanding individual dietary needs, and remaining attuned to the dog's overall health. By providing a diverse and nutritionally complete diet, pet owners can contribute to the well-being and happiness of their canine companions.

Choosing the Right Low-Fat Ingredients

3.1 Lean Protein Sources

Protein, an indispensable component of a dog's diet, plays a vital role in various physiological functions, including muscle development, immune support, and overall health. Incorporating lean protein sources ensures that dogs receive the necessary amino acids without an excess of fat, promoting optimal well-being. Here are some excellent lean protein sources for dogs:

1. Chicken Breast:
Skinless, boneless chicken breast is a lean and easily digestible protein source. It provides essential amino acids, making it a staple in many dog diets. Boiling or baking chicken breast without added fats ensures a nutritious and low-fat protein option.

2. Turkey:
Similar to chicken, lean turkey meat is an excellent source of protein. Ground turkey or lean turkey cuts offer variety in taste while providing the necessary nutrients. It's important to avoid using processed

turkey products that may contain added fats or seasonings.

3. Fish:

Certain fish, such as cod, haddock, and flounder, are lean protein sources rich in omega-3 fatty acids. These fatty acids contribute to skin and coat health while supporting joint function. It's crucial to ensure that fish is cooked thoroughly and bone-free before serving.

4. Lean Beef:

Lean cuts of meat, like sirloin or tenderloin, offer protein without exorbitant fat. Trimming visible fat before cooking minimizes the fat content. Ground beef labeled as 90% lean or higher is also a suitable option when cooked without added fats.

5. Eggs:

Eggs, particularly egg whites, are a highly digestible and protein-rich option. They provide a complete source of amino acids. Cooking eggs thoroughly is important to avoid potential issues with biotin absorption.

6. Venison:

Venison, the meat of deer, is a lean and novel protein source for dogs. It offers a different taste profile and is often well-tolerated by dogs with food sensitivities. Ensure that venison is sourced from reputable and safe suppliers.

7. Pork Tenderloin:
Pork tenderloin is a lean cut of pork that can give protein to a canine's eating regimen. Trim away visible fat before cooking to maintain a low-fat profile. It's crucial to avoid processed pork products high in salt and preservatives.

8. Lamb:
Lean cuts of lamb, such as loin or leg, can be included in a dog's diet in moderation. Lamb is a good source of protein and essential nutrients. As with other meats, trimming excess fat is essential.

9. Cottage Cheese:
Cottage cheese is a dairy-based protein source that is low in fat. It provides dogs with protein and calcium. Opt for low-fat or fat-free varieties and feed in moderation, especially if a dog is lactose intolerant.

10. Lean Venison:
Venison, similar to other game meats, is often lean and offers a novel protein source. It can be suitable for dogs

with food allergies or sensitivities. Ensure that venison is prepared and cooked thoroughly.

When incorporating lean protein sources into a dog's diet, it's crucial to consider the dog's individual needs, such as breed, size, and health status. Additionally, consulting with a veterinarian helps tailor the diet to meet specific nutritional requirements and ensures that the dog receives a well-rounded and balanced nutritional profile.

3.2 Healthy Carbohydrates for Sustained Energy

Carbohydrates serve as a primary source of energy for dogs, providing the fuel necessary for various bodily functions and activities. Opting for healthy carbohydrates ensures sustained energy levels, supports overall health, and contributes to a well-balanced canine diet. Here are some excellent sources of healthy carbohydrates for dogs:

1. Brown Rice:
Brown rice is a whole grain that provides complex carbohydrates, fiber, and essential nutrients. It offers sustained energy release, making it an ideal component of a dog's diet. Ensure that the rice is thoroughly cooked for easy digestion.

2. Sweet Potatoes:
Sweet potatoes are rich in complex carbohydrates, fiber, and vitamins. They offer a natural sweetness and are easily digestible. Including sweet potatoes in a dog's diet contributes to sustained energy levels and supports digestive health.

3. Quinoa:

Quinoa is a complete protein source that also contains complex carbohydrates. It gives canines a scope of fundamental amino acids and is sans gluten. Cooked quinoa can be added to a dog's meals to enhance nutritional diversity.

4. Oatmeal:

Oatmeal is a wholesome and easily digestible carbohydrate option for dogs. It contains soluble fiber, promoting digestive health, and releases energy gradually. Ensure that oatmeal is plain and free from added sugars or flavorings.

5. Barley:

Barley is a whole grain rich in fiber, vitamins, and minerals. It offers sustained energy and contributes to digestive well-being. Cooked barley can be included in a dog's diet as a source of complex carbohydrates.

6. Pumpkin:

Pumpkin is not only a great source of fiber but also provides carbohydrates for energy. It is easily digestible and can be included in a dog's diet to support digestive regularity. Opt for plain, canned pumpkin without added sugars or spices.

7. Whole Wheat:

Whole wheat products, such as whole wheat pasta or whole wheat bread, can contribute to a dog's carbohydrate intake. These should be fed in moderation, and it's essential to avoid products with added sugars or unhealthy additives.

8. Legumes (Chickpeas, Lentils):

Legumes like chickpeas and lentils offer a combination of protein and complex carbohydrates. They are rich in fiber, promoting digestive health, and can be included in a dog's diet either as a main ingredient or as part of a balanced meal.

9. Peas:

Peas are a nutrient-rich vegetable that provides carbohydrates, fiber, and essential vitamins. They can be included in a dog's diet as part of a balanced meal or as a treat. Fresh or frozen peas are preferable to canned options.

10. Carrots:

Carrots are a crunchy and nutritious vegetable that contains natural sugars and fiber. They are a healthy carbohydrate option that can be used as a snack or added to a dog's meals.

When incorporating healthy carbohydrates into a dog's diet, it's important to consider the individual needs of the dog, such as age, activity level, and health status. Additionally, consulting with a veterinarian ensures that the carbohydrate sources chosen align with the dog's nutritional requirements, contributing to sustained energy levels and overall well-being.

3.3 Essential Fats in Moderation

While fats are a crucial component of a dog's diet, their intake must be managed judiciously to strike a balance between providing essential nutrients and avoiding potential health issues. Essential fats play a vital role in a dog's overall well-being, contributing to various physiological functions. Here's an exploration of incorporating essential fats in moderation into a dog's diet:

1. Omega-3 Fatty Acids:
Omega-3 fatty acids, found in fish oil, flaxseed, and certain fish varieties, are essential for dogs. They support coat and skin health, reduce inflammation, and may contribute to joint function. Incorporating these fats in moderation enhances the nutritional profile of a dog's diet.

2. Fish as a Source of Essential Fats:
Certain fish, such as salmon and mackerel, are rich in omega-3 fatty acids. Including these fish in a dog's diet can provide essential fats along with protein. It's essential to cook fish thoroughly to eliminate the risk of parasites.

3. Flaxseed Oil:

Flaxseed oil is a plant-based source of omega-3 fatty acids. It can be added to a dog's food in moderation to promote healthy skin and coat. Keep in mind that moderation is key, as excessive fat intake can lead to digestive issues.

4. Coconut Oil:

Coconut oil contains medium-chain triglycerides (MCTs) that can contribute to a dog's energy levels. While it's beneficial in moderation, it's crucial to avoid overfeeding, as coconut oil is calorie-dense. Start with small amounts and monitor your dog's response.

5. Avocado:

Avocado is a source of monounsaturated fats, which can contribute to a dog's overall fat intake. While it provides healthy fats, avocado should be fed in moderation, and the pit and skin must be removed, as they contain substances that can be toxic to dogs.

6. Balancing Fat Intake:

Moderation in fat intake is critical to prevent obesity and related health issues. Dogs with specific health conditions, such as pancreatitis, may require even stricter fat control. Consult with a veterinarian to determine the appropriate fat levels for your dog's individual needs.

7. Essential Fats for Brain Health:
Fats play a role in supporting cognitive function and brain health in dogs. Including essential fats in moderation can contribute to mental acuity, especially in aging dogs. It's essential to balance fat intake with other nutrients to maintain overall health.

8. Checking Labels for Fat Content:
When selecting commercial dog food or treats, it's crucial to check labels for fat content. Opt for products that provide essential fats in appropriate proportions while avoiding those with excessive saturated or unhealthy fats.

9. Weight Management:
Monitoring a dog's weight is integral to maintaining health. Essential fats contribute to overall well-being but should be factored into the dog's total caloric intake. Adjust the diet as needed to prevent weight gain or loss.

10. Individualized Nutrition Plans:

Each dog is unique, and their nutritional needs can vary based on factors such as breed, age, and health status. Work closely with a veterinarian to create an individualized nutrition plan that considers the dog's specific requirements.

Essential fats are valuable contributors to a dog's health, but moderation is key. By selecting healthy fat sources and monitoring intake, pet owners can enhance their canine companions' well-being, promoting vibrant skin, glossy coats, and overall vitality. Always consult with a veterinarian to tailor dietary recommendations to the specific needs of your dog.

Homemade Low-Fat Dog Food Recipes

4.1 Vet-Approved Recipes

1. Chicken and Rice Delight:
Ingredients:

- Chicken breast, cooked and shredded
- Brown rice, cooked
- Carrots, finely chopped
- Peas, frozen or fresh
- Fish oil (as a source of omega-3 fatty acids)

Directions:
1. Mix all ingredients together, ensuring the chicken is thoroughly cooked. Serve once cooled.

2. Beef and Vegetable Stew:
Ingredients:

- Lean ground beef
- Sweet potatoes, diced
- Green beans, chopped
- Carrots, sliced
- Beef broth (low-sodium)

Directions:

1. Brown the beef, add vegetables and broth, and simmer until vegetables are tender.

3. Turkey and Quinoa Feast:

Ingredients:

- Ground turkey
- Quinoa, cooked
- Spinach, finely chopped
- Blueberries (as a treat)
- Coconut oil (in moderation)

Directions:

1. Cook turkey, mix with quinoa, add spinach, and top with a few blueberries.

4. Salmon and Sweet Potato Surprise:

Ingredients:

- Salmon filet, cooked and flaked
- Sweet potatoes, mashed
- Broccoli, steamed
- Chia seeds (for added nutrients)

Directions:

1. Combine flaked salmon, mashed sweet potatoes, and steamed broccoli. Sprinkle it with chia seeds.

5. Egg and Spinach Omelet:

Ingredients:

- Eggs
- Spinach, chopped
- Carrots, grated
- Cottage cheese (optional)

Directions:

1. Whisk eggs, add spinach and carrots, and cook as an omelet. Add cottage cheese if desired.

6. Lamb and Barley Stew:

Ingredients:

- Lean lamb meat, diced
- Barley, cooked
- Peas, frozen or fresh
- Pumpkin, cubed
- Turmeric (as an anti-inflammatory)

Directions:

1. Cook lamb, add cooked barley, peas, pumpkin, and a pinch of turmeric.

7. Venison and Rice Medley:

Ingredients:

- Venison, cooked and shredded
- White rice, cooked
- Carrots, finely chopped
- Blueberries (as a treat)
- Flaxseed oil (as a wellspring of omega-3 unsaturated fats)

Directions:

1. Combine shredded venison, cooked rice, chopped carrots, and a drizzle of flaxseed oil. Add a few blueberries as a treat.

8. Pork and Potato Fiesta:

Ingredients:

- Lean pork, cooked and diced
- Potatoes, mashed
- Green peas, steamed
- Apples, diced
- Cinnamon (for flavor)

Directions:

1. Mix cooked pork with mashed potatoes, add steamed peas, diced apples, and a dash of cinnamon.

9. Duck and Lentil Delicacy:

Ingredients:

- Duck breast, cooked and sliced
- Lentils, cooked
- Carrots, grated
- Blueberries (as a treat)
- Olive oil (in moderation)

Directions:

1. Combine sliced duck, cooked lentils, grated carrots, and a drizzle of olive oil. Add a few blueberries as a treat.

10. Chicken Liver and Pumpkin Casserole:

Ingredients:

- Chicken liver, cooked and chopped
- Pumpkin, pureed
- Green beans, chopped
- Cranberries (as a treat)
- Yogurt (plain, as a topping)

Directions:

1. Mix chopped chicken liver, pumpkin puree, chopped green beans. Top with a dollop of plain yogurt and a few cranberries.

11. Sardine and Quinoa Surprise:

Ingredients:

- Canned sardines in water, drained
- Quinoa, cooked
- Spinach, finely chopped
- Carrots, grated
- Parsley (for freshness)

Directions:

1. Mix drained sardines, cooked quinoa, chopped spinach, grated carrots, and chopped parsley.

12. Chicken and Blueberry Bliss:

Ingredients:

- Ground chicken
- Blueberries
- Brown rice, cooked
- Zucchini, grated
- Coconut oil (in moderation)

Directions:

1. Cook ground chicken, mix with blueberries, cooked brown rice, and grated zucchini. Drizzle with a little coconut oil.

Remember to adjust portion sizes based on your dog's size, weight, and activity level. Additionally, consult with your veterinarian to ensure these recipes align with your dog's specific dietary needs.

4.2 Cooking Techniques for Retaining Nutrient Value

Preparing homemade dog food involves careful consideration of cooking techniques to retain the maximum nutritional value of the ingredients. The right cooking methods ensure that your canine companion receives the essential nutrients from their meals. Here are cooking techniques that help preserve the nutrient content in dog food:

1. Steaming:
Steaming is a gentle cooking method that helps retain the natural flavors and nutrients in vegetables. Steam vegetables like carrots, broccoli, or green beans until they are tender but still crisp. This method minimizes nutrient loss through water and heat exposure.

2. Boiling:
Boiling is a simple method that can help preserve nutrient content. When cooking meats or grains, use the minimum amount of water necessary and consider using the water as a part of the meal to retain water-soluble vitamins and minerals.

3. Blanching:
Blanching involves briefly immersing vegetables in boiling water and then rapidly cooling them. This method helps preserve the color, texture, and nutritional value of vegetables. It's particularly useful for vegetables that can be served to dogs in their raw state.

4. Baking:
Baking is a dry heat method that can be suitable for cooking meats and certain vegetables. It allows for the retention of flavors and nutrients without excessive nutrient loss. Use minimal fats or oils when baking to keep the meal healthy.

5. Microwaving:
Microwaving is a quick and efficient cooking method that retains nutrients well, especially when cooking vegetables. Use microwave-safe containers, and cover them to minimize nutrient loss through evaporation.

6. Slow Cooking:
Slow cooking at lower temperatures over an extended period can help preserve nutrients. This method is particularly useful for preparing stews or casseroles

with meats, vegetables, and grains. Ensure that the ingredients are cooked thoroughly.

7. Raw Feeding:
Raw feeding involves serving uncooked ingredients like raw meat, bones, and vegetables. While it requires careful planning to ensure a balanced diet, feeding some ingredients raw can help preserve their natural nutrients.

8. Minimizing Overcooking:
Avoid overcooking ingredients, especially meats, as prolonged exposure to high heat can lead to nutrient degradation. Cook meats until they are safe for consumption but not excessively well-done.

9. Using Cooking Liquids:
When preparing homemade dog food, consider incorporating cooking liquids, such as broth or water, into the final meal. This helps retain water-soluble vitamins and minerals that may leach into the liquid during cooking.

10. Avoiding Excessive Fats:
While fats are essential for dogs, excessive fat during cooking may lead to nutrient loss. Use cooking

methods that minimize the need for added fats, such as grilling or baking without excessive oil.

11. Proper Storage:
After cooking, store dog food in airtight containers in the refrigerator or freezer. Proper storage helps maintain the freshness and nutritional value of the food.

12. Balancing Raw and Cooked Ingredients:
Combining both raw and cooked ingredients in your dog's diet can provide a variety of nutrients. Ensure that raw components are safe and sourced from reputable suppliers.

4.3 Transitioning to Homemade Diets Safely

Transitioning your dog to a homemade diet requires careful planning and a gradual approach to ensure their nutritional needs are met. Sudden changes to a dog's diet can lead to digestive upset, so it's essential to follow a systematic process. Here's a guide to safely transition your dog to a homemade diet:

1. Consult Your Veterinarian:
Before making any dietary changes, consult with your veterinarian. They can assess your dog's health, discuss specific dietary requirements, and provide guidance on appropriate nutrient levels.

2. Research and Plan:
Invest time in researching balanced and nutritionally complete homemade dog food recipes. Consider factors such as your dog's breed, size, age, and any specific health concerns.

3. Start Slowly:
Begin by incorporating small amounts of homemade food alongside your dog's regular diet. Gradually

increase the proportion of homemade food while reducing the commercial diet over several days or weeks.

4. Monitor for Digestive Changes:
Keep a close eye on your dog's stool, appetite, and overall behavior during the transition. If you notice any signs of digestive upset, such as diarrhea or vomiting, slow down the transition process.

5. Maintain Consistency:
Consistency is key during the transition. Use the same protein sources, grains, and vegetables for a few days before introducing new ingredients. This helps your dog's digestive system adapt gradually.

6. Balanced Diet:
Ensure the homemade diet is well-balanced and includes a variety of proteins, carbohydrates, healthy fats, and vegetables. Aim for a diverse nutrient profile to meet your dog's nutritional needs.

7. Include Supplements as Needed:
Depending on your dog's individual requirements, your veterinarian may recommend supplements such as calcium, omega-3 fatty acids, or specific vitamins.

Integrate these supplements into the homemade diet as advised.

8. Be Mindful of Allergies:

If your dog has known food allergies or sensitivities, choose ingredients that are less likely to trigger adverse reactions. Monitor for any signs of allergic reactions during the transition.

9. Watch for Weight Changes:

Adjust the portion sizes of homemade food based on your dog's weight and activity level. Monitor for any weight loss or gain and adjust the diet accordingly.

10. Hydration is Crucial:

Ensure your dog has access to fresh water at all times. A homemade diet may have different moisture content than commercial kibble, so hydration is essential for overall health.

11. Regular Vet Check-ups:

Schedule regular veterinary check-ups to assess your dog's overall health and address any concerns. Your veterinarian can provide ongoing guidance on your dog's homemade diet.

12. Seek Professional Advice:
If you're unsure about any aspect of the transition or your dog's nutritional needs, seek professional advice promptly. Your veterinarian or a canine nutritionist can provide valuable insights.

13. Transitioning to Raw Diets:
If considering a raw diet, take extra precautions to handle and store raw ingredients safely. Consult with your veterinarian to ensure the raw diet is nutritionally complete and safe for your dog.

14. Stay Patient and Flexible:
Each dog is unique, and the transition process may vary. Stay patient, be flexible with your approach, and make adjustments based on your dog's individual response.

Transitioning to a homemade diet for your dog can be a rewarding and healthful choice when done with careful planning and monitoring. By following these steps and working closely with your veterinarian, you can provide your canine companion with a nutritionally balanced and wholesome diet tailored to their individual needs.

Feeding Strategies and Portion Control

5.1 Meal Frequency and Timing

Establishing a proper meal frequency and timing is crucial to maintaining your dog's health and well-being. The right feeding schedule ensures that your canine companion receives the necessary nutrients at regular intervals throughout the day. Here's a guide to help you determine the most suitable meal frequency and timing for your dog:

1. Consider Age and Life Stage:

Puppies: Young puppies typically require more frequent meals due to their rapid growth. Feed them three to four times a day until they are around six months old, then gradually transition to two meals a day.

Adult Dogs: Most grown-up canines really do well with two dinners each day. Nonetheless, individual requirements might shift in view of variables like variety, size, and movement level.

Senior Dogs: As canines age, their digestion might dial back. Consider maintaining two meals per day or adjusting the portion sizes based on your senior dog's energy requirements.

2. Divide Daily Portion into Meals:

Determine the total daily amount of food recommended for your dog based on their weight, activity level, and health status.

Divide this daily portion into the desired number of meals. For example, if feeding twice a day, split the daily amount into two equal portions.

3. Stick to a Consistent Schedule:

Dogs thrive on routine. Try to feed your dog at the same time each day to establish a consistent schedule.

Consistency helps regulate your dog's digestion, makes potty training easier, and contributes to a sense of security.

4. Avoid Free Feeding:

Free feeding (leaving food out for your dog to eat at their leisure) may lead to overeating and weight gain.

A structured feeding schedule helps monitor your dog's food intake and makes it easier to identify changes in appetite.

5. Monitor Activity Levels:

Consider your dog's activity level when determining portion sizes and feeding frequency.

More active dogs may benefit from additional meals or larger portions, while less active dogs may require smaller, more frequent meals.

6. Adjust for Medical Conditions:

A few ailments, like diabetes or gastrointestinal issues, may require explicit taking care of timetables.

Consult with your veterinarian to determine the most appropriate meal frequency and timing based on your dog's health needs.

7. Post-Exercise Meals:

Consider feeding your dog after exercise to replenish energy stores and promote muscle recovery.

Wait at least 30 minutes to an hour after vigorous exercise before offering a meal to avoid potential stomach upset.

8. Morning and Evening Feedings:

Many dog owners find success with morning and evening feedings. This allows your dog to start the day with energy and ensures they have a satisfied stomach before bedtime.

9. Avoid Feeding Immediately Before Exercise:

Feeding right before exercise may lead to discomfort or digestive issues. Aim to feed your dog at least an hour before physical activity.

10. Special Considerations for Raw Diets:

If feeding a raw diet, ensure that raw meat and other perishable ingredients are handled and stored safely.

Divide the daily raw food portion into meals and follow similar guidelines for feeding frequency.

11. Observe and Adjust:

Monitor your dog's weight, body condition, and overall health regularly.

Change segment sizes and take care of recurrence in view of your canine's singular requirements and any progressions in action level.

12. Hydration is Key:

Always provide access to fresh water. Hydration is essential for digestion, nutrient absorption, and overall well-being.

5.2 Monitoring Your Dog's Weight and Health

Keeping a sound weight is essential for your canine's general prosperity. Regular monitoring of your dog's weight and health allows you to identify any potential issues early on, ensuring that your furry friend enjoys a happy and active life. Here's a comprehensive guide on how to effectively monitor your dog's weight and health:

1. Weighing Your Dog:
Use a Reliable Scale: Invest in a reliable scale to weigh your dog accurately. If your dog is small, you can step on the scale first, note your weight, and then pick up your dog, subtracting your weight from the total.

Establish a Routine: Weigh your dog regularly, ideally once a month. Consistency in timing and conditions (such as before meals or at the same time of day) helps provide accurate tracking.

Keep a Record: Maintain a record of your dog's weight over time. A consistent log allows you to identify trends and detect any significant changes.

2. Body Condition Scoring:

Learn the Basics: Familiarize yourself with body condition scoring systems provided by veterinarians or pet health organizations. These systems typically assess factors like ribs, waist, and overall muscle mass.

Regular Assessment: Conduct regular visual and tactile assessments of your dog's body condition. A healthy weight should feature a well-defined waist and the ability to feel, but not see, the ribs.

3. Behavioral and Energy Changes:

Monitor Activity Levels: Note any significant changes in your dog's energy levels or activity. Sudden lethargy or excessive restlessness can be indicators of health issues.

Watch for Changes in Appetite: Changes in eating habits, such as a sudden increase or decrease in appetite, may signal health concerns. Consult your veterinarian if you notice any drastic changes.

4. Regular Veterinary Check-ups:

Schedule Routine Visits: Regular veterinary check-ups are essential for preventive care. These visits allow your veterinarian to assess your dog's overall health, address concerns, and offer guidance on nutrition and weight management.

Dental Health Checks: Oral health is a crucial component of overall well-being. Schedule regular dental check-ups and maintain good dental hygiene practices.

5. Parasite Prevention:

Implement Regular Parasite Control: Parasites, such as fleas and worms, can impact your dog's health and weight. Follow a veterinarian-recommended parasite prevention plan to keep your dog healthy.

Monitor Stool Consistency: Changes in stool consistency can be indicators of digestive issues or parasites. Regularly inspect your dog's stool for any abnormalities.

6. Routine Blood Work:

Consider Routine Blood Tests: Depending on your dog's age and health status, your veterinarian may recommend routine blood tests. These tests can provide valuable insights into your dog's internal health.

Screen for Common Health Issues: Blood tests can help screen for common health issues, including organ function, thyroid levels, and metabolic conditions.

7. Weight Management Plans:
Work with Your Veterinarian: If your dog needs to gain or lose weight, consult with your veterinarian to create a customized weight management plan.

Adjust Diet and Exercise: Modify your dog's diet and exercise routine based on your veterinarian's recommendations. This may involve changes in portion sizes, dietary composition, or activity levels.

8. Be Mindful of Breed Characteristics:
Consider Breed-Specific Traits: Some breeds are naturally leaner or heavier. Be aware of your dog's breed characteristics and consult with your veterinarian to determine the ideal weight range.

9. Senior Dog Health Monitoring:
Adapt to Aging Needs: As dogs age, their nutritional and health needs may change. Work closely with your veterinarian to adapt their diet, exercise, and health monitoring strategies.

Joint Health Considerations: Senior dogs may be prone to joint issues. Monitor for signs of stiffness or discomfort, and discuss joint health supplements with your veterinarian.

10. Maintain a Balanced Diet:

Choose Nutrient-Rich Foods: Select a high-quality dog food that meets your dog's specific nutritional requirements. Consult with your veterinarian for guidance on appropriate portion sizes.

Avoid Excessive Treats: Limit treats and avoid overfeeding. Excessive treats can contribute to weight gain and nutritional imbalances.

Monitoring your dog's weight and health is a proactive approach to ensure they lead a happy, healthy life. Regular assessments, veterinary check-ups, and a keen awareness of changes in behavior or physical condition enable you to address any concerns promptly. Remember, your veterinarian is a valuable partner in maintaining your dog's optimal health, offering tailored advice and guidance based on your dog's individual needs.

5.3 Adjusting Portions Based on Activity Levels

Tailoring your dog's food portions to their activity level is a fundamental aspect of responsible pet care. Dogs with varying activity levels have different energy requirements, and adjusting their portions accordingly ensures they receive the right balance of nutrients. Here's a guide on how to adapt your dog's portions based on their activity levels:

1. Understanding Activity Levels:

Low Activity Level:
Dogs with low activity levels, such as seniors or those with health concerns, may have reduced energy needs. They require less calories to keep a solid weight.

Moderate Activity Level:
Most adult dogs fall into this category. Regular walks, playtime, and moderate exercise characterize their routine. Adjust portions to match their energy expenditure.

High Activity Level:
Working dogs, highly active breeds, or dogs involved in competitive sports have high energy needs. They require increased caloric intake to support their active lifestyle.

2. Consult with Your Veterinarian:
Individualized Advice:
Consult with your veterinarian to determine your dog's appropriate activity level and nutritional requirements. Breed, age, health status, and other factors influence their recommendations.

Special Considerations:
Dogs with specific health conditions or those in unique life stages (puppies, seniors) may have special dietary needs. Your veterinarian can give customized guidance.

3. Energy Expenditure Calculation:
Calorie Calculations:
Calculate your dog's daily caloric needs based on factors like size, age, and activity level. Your veterinarian or pet nutritionist can assist in determining the appropriate daily caloric intake.

Weight Monitoring:
Regularly monitor your dog's weight. Adjust portions if you notice weight gain or loss, ensuring they stay within the healthy weight range.

4. Portion Control Guidelines:
Low Activity Dogs:
For dogs with low activity levels, provide smaller portions to prevent excess calorie intake. Choose a high-quality, nutrient-dense food to meet their nutritional needs without excess calories.

Moderate Activity Dogs:
Offer portions that align with their moderate energy expenditure. Dividing their daily food into two meals provides sustained energy throughout the day.

High Activity Dogs:
Dogs with high activity levels may require larger portions or a diet with a higher calorie density. Frequent meals can help meet their increased energy demands.

5. Monitor and Adjust:
Regular Observation:

Screen your canine's body condition consistently. Adjust portions if you observe changes in weight, such as gradual weight gain or loss.

Adapt to Seasonal Changes:
Dogs may have varying activity levels based on weather conditions. Adjust portions seasonally to accommodate changes in exercise routines.

6. Consider Treats and Training Rewards:
Caloric Contribution:
Factor in the calories from treats and training rewards. Be mindful of the overall caloric intake to avoid unintentional overfeeding.

Choose Healthy Treats:
Opt for healthy, low-calorie treats or use a portion of your dog's regular food as rewards during training sessions.

7. Hydration and Nutrient Balance:
Ensure Adequate Hydration:
Regardless of activity level, always provide access to fresh water. Proper hydration is essential for overall health and digestion.

Balanced Nutrient Intake:

While adjusting portions, maintain a balanced nutrient intake. Ensure your dog's diet provides essential proteins, fats, vitamins, and minerals.

8. Customizing Diets for Working Dogs:

Special Considerations:

Working dogs, such as those in search and rescue or police work, may have unique nutritional needs. Collaborate with your veterinarian to create a diet that supports their demanding work.

High-Calorie Diets:

Consider high-calorie diets or supplements for dogs with intense physical demands. These should be administered under the guidance of a veterinarian.

9. Transition Periods:

Gradual Adjustments:

When changing your dog's activity level or adjusting portions, do so gradually. Sudden changes can lead to digestive upset.

Monitor Response:

Observe how your dog responds to the adjusted portions. Behavioral changes, energy levels, and overall well-being provide valuable feedback.

Supplements for Pancreatitis Management

6.1 Omega-3 Fatty Acids

Omega-3 unsaturated fats are a gathering of polyunsaturated fats that assume a significant part in keeping up with your canine's general wellbeing. These essential fatty acids, particularly eicosapentaenoic acid (EPA) and docosahexaenoic acid (DHA), offer a range of benefits for your canine companion. Here's a comprehensive overview of Omega-3 fatty acids and their significance in your dog's diet:

1. Sources of Omega-3 Fatty Acids:
Fish Oil: Rich in EPA and DHA, fish oil derived from fatty fish like salmon, mackerel, and sardines is a common supplement.

Algal Oil: Suitable for dogs with fish allergies, algal oil is derived from algae and provides a plant-based source of DHA.

Flaxseed: Flaxseed a plant-based wellspring of alpha-linolenic corrosive (ALA), a forerunner to EPA and DHA. However, dogs may not efficiently convert ALA to the active forms.

2. Benefits of Omega-3 Fatty Acids for Dogs:

Joint Health: Omega-3s have anti-inflammatory properties that can help manage joint conditions such as arthritis, promoting mobility and reducing discomfort.

Skin and Coat Health: EPA and DHA contribute to a healthy, shiny coat and can alleviate skin conditions such as allergies and dry, itchy skin.

Heart Health: Omega-3s support cardiovascular health by reducing the risk of heart disease and maintaining proper blood flow.

Cognitive Function: DHA, in particular, plays a vital role in brain development and cognitive function, making it beneficial for puppies and senior dogs.

Immune System Support: Omega-3s have anti-inflammatory effects that support a robust immune system, helping the body fight off infections and diseases.

3. Picking the Right Omega-3 Enhancement:

Quality Matters: Opt for high-quality, reputable supplements to ensure they are free from contaminants and provide the stated levels of EPA and DHA.

Dosage Considerations: Consult with your veterinarian to determine the appropriate dosage based on your dog's size, age, Stand specific health needs.

4.Integrating Omega-3s into Your Canine's Eating regimen:

Commercial Dog Food: Some high-quality commercial dog foods are enriched with Omega-3 fatty acids. Check the label for details.

Supplements: If your dog's diet lacks sufficient Omega-3s, consider adding fish oil or algal oil supplements. These are available in liquid or capsule form.

Natural Sources: Include fatty fish in your dog's diet, such as salmon or mackerel, to naturally boost their Omega-3 intake.

5. Caution with Fish Oil:

Watch for Allergies: While fish oil is beneficial for most dogs, some may be allergic to certain fish. Screen your canine for any indications of antagonistic responses.

Balance Omega-3 and Omega-6: Ensure a balanced ratio of Omega-3 to Omega-6 fatty acids in your dog's diet. Omega-6s are found in many oils, and an excessive imbalance can lead to inflammation.

6. Consulting with Your Veterinarian:

Individualized Recommendations: Your veterinarian can provide personalized advice on the optimal dosage and sources of Omega-3s based on your dog's health status.

Monitoring Health Conditions: If your dog has specific health conditions, such as allergies, arthritis, or skin issues, Omega-3 supplementation may be tailored to address these concerns.

7. Transitioning to a Homemade Diet:

Balancing Nutrients: If you're considering a homemade diet, work with your veterinarian to ensure it is well-balanced, and consider including natural sources of Omega-3s.

8. Monitoring Your Dog's Response:

Observe Changes: As you introduce Omega-3 supplements or adjust the diet, observe your dog for positive changes in coat condition, mobility, and overall well-being.

Adjust as Needed: If you notice any adverse effects or if your dog's health needs change, consult with your veterinarian to adjust the Omega-3 supplementation accordingly.

6.2 Digestive Enzymes

Digestive enzymes are essential compounds that play a vital role in breaking down food into nutrients that the body can absorb and utilize. In dogs, as in humans, these enzymes contribute to effective digestion and nutrient absorption. Here's a comprehensive guide to understanding digestive enzymes in dogs:

1. Kinds of Stomach related Catalysts:

Amylase: Separates starches into less difficult sugars.

Lipase: Helps in the absorption of fats, separating them into unsaturated fats and glycerol.

Protease: Separates proteins into amino acids.

Cellulase: Helps with separating cellulose, a perplexing starch found in plant cell walls.

2. Wellsprings of Stomach related Compounds:

Endogenous Compounds: Created by the canine's body, principally in the pancreas and small digestive system.

Exogenous Enzymes: Obtained from external sources, such as certain raw foods or commercial enzyme supplements.

3. The Role of Digestive Enzymes in Canine Health:

Nutrient Absorption: Enzymes facilitate the breakdown of food into smaller, absorbable components, allowing the body to extract and utilize essential nutrients.

Digestive Efficiency: Adequate enzyme activity supports efficient digestion, reducing the risk of gastrointestinal discomfort and issues such as bloating or gas.

Energy Production: By breaking down nutrients, enzymes contribute to the production of energy that fuels various bodily functions.

4. Conditions Requiring Digestive Enzyme Support:

Exocrine Pancreatic Insufficiency (EPI): In EPI, the pancreas doesn't produce enough digestive enzymes, leading to malabsorption of nutrients. Enzyme supplementation is often prescribed.

Sensitive Stomachs: Dogs with digestive sensitivities or food intolerances may benefit from additional enzyme support.

Aging Dogs: Older dogs may experience a natural decline in enzyme production, making supplementation beneficial for maintaining optimal digestion.

5. Regular Wellsprings of Stomach related Chemicals:

Raw Foods: Raw, unprocessed foods contain natural enzymes that can support digestion. Raw diets, when well-balanced, may contribute to enzyme intake.

Sprouted Foods: Certain sprouted grains, vegetables, and legumes are rich in enzymes and can be included in a dog's diet.

6. Commercial Digestive Enzyme Supplements:

Available Forms: Digestive enzyme supplements come in various forms, including powders, capsules, and chewable tablets.

Consultation with Veterinarian: If considering supplementation, consult with your veterinarian to ensure the choice aligns with your dog's specific needs.

7. Considerations for Usage:

Meal Timing: Enzyme supplements are typically administered with meals to aid in the digestion of specific nutrients.

Dosage Guidelines: Follow recommended dosage guidelines provided by your veterinarian or the product manufacturer.

Monitoring Response: Observe your dog for any changes in digestion, stool consistency, and overall well-being after introducing enzyme supplements.

8. Potential Benefits of Digestive Enzyme Supplementation:

Reduced Gastrointestinal Discomfort: Enzyme supplements may alleviate symptoms such as bloating, gas, and diarrhea, especially in dogs with digestive issues.

Improved Nutrient Absorption: Enhanced digestion can lead to better absorption of nutrients, supporting overall health.

Optimized Weight Management: Efficient digestion may contribute to maintaining a healthy weight in dogs.

9. Caution and Monitoring:

Allergic Reactions: Monitor for any signs of allergic reactions to supplements, such as itching, swelling, or digestive upset.

Underlying Health Conditions: Before starting any supplementation, rule out underlying health conditions that may require specific interventions.

10. Natural Ways to Support Digestive Enzymes:

Prebiotics and Probiotics: These promote a healthy gut environment, supporting the activity of digestive enzymes.

Balanced Diet: A well-balanced diet with high-quality ingredients can naturally provide a spectrum of enzymes.

11. Consult with Your Veterinarian:

Individualized Guidance: Your veterinarian can assess your dog's specific needs and provide individualized recommendations for enzyme supplementation or dietary adjustments.

Understanding the role of digestive enzymes in your dog's health allows you to make informed decisions about their diet and supplementation. Working closely with your veterinarian ensures that any changes to your dog's diet align with their unique health requirements.

6.3 Veterinary Recommendations

Veterinary recommendations are the cornerstone of proactive and preventive care for your canine companion. Regular check-ups and guidance from a trusted veterinarian play a crucial role in ensuring your dog's well-being. Here's a comprehensive guide on the key aspects of veterinary recommendations for optimal canine health:

1. Routine Wellness Examinations:

Frequency: Schedule regular wellness examinations at least once a year for adult dogs, and more frequently for puppies, seniors, or those with specific health concerns.

Comprehensive Assessment: Wellness exams encompass a thorough physical examination, dental evaluation, and discussion of your dog's behavior, diet, and lifestyle.

2. Vaccinations and Preventive Care:

Tailored Vaccination Schedule: Your veterinarian will create a vaccination plan tailored to your dog's age, lifestyle, and risk factors.

Parasite Prevention: Regular administration of preventive medications protects against fleas, ticks, heartworms, and intestinal parasites.

3. Nutritional Guidance:

Dietary Recommendations: Your veterinarian can provide advice on selecting the right commercial dog food or guide you in preparing a nutritionally balanced homemade diet.

Weight Management: Maintain a healthy weight for your dog through portion control and appropriate exercise.

4. Dental Care:

Importance of Dental Health: Dental issues can impact overall health. Your veterinarian may recommend dental cleanings, dental diets, or dental care routines at home.

Periodic Dental Check-ups: Regular dental check-ups can identify and address dental problems early on.

5. Behavioral Consultations:

Understanding Behavior: If you notice changes in your dog's behavior, seek guidance from your veterinarian. They can assess whether there are underlying health issues or behavioral concerns that need attention.

Training and Socialization: Your veterinarian can offer recommendations on training, socialization, and addressing behavioral challenges.

6. Senior Dog Care:

Increased Frequency of Check-ups: Senior dogs often require more frequent veterinary visits. Regular screenings for conditions like arthritis, kidney disease, and cognitive decline become essential.

Nutritional Adjustments: Dietary changes may be necessary for senior dogs. Your veterinarian can recommend appropriate senior diets and supplements.

7. Diagnostic Testing:

Blood Work and Urinalysis: Periodic diagnostic tests, especially as your dog ages, help identify and monitor conditions such as kidney disease, diabetes, or liver issues.

Imaging Studies: X-rays, ultrasounds, or other imaging studies may be recommended to investigate specific health concerns.

8. Spaying and Neutering:

Timing and Considerations: Discuss the optimal timing for spaying or neutering your dog with your veterinarian. Factors such as breed, size, and overall health play a role in these decisions.

9. Emergency Preparedness:

Emergency Contact Information: Keep your veterinarian's contact information easily accessible, and be aware of emergency veterinary services in your area.

First Aid Kit: Maintain a basic first aid kit for your dog, and know how to respond to common emergencies.

10. Ongoing Communication:

Open Dialogue: Foster open communication with your veterinarian. Discuss any concerns, changes in behavior, or potential health issues promptly.

Follow-Up Visits: Follow-up visits are crucial after treatments or surgeries to monitor your dog's recovery.

11. Weight and Exercise Management:

Regular Exercise: Your veterinarian can guide you on appropriate exercise for your dog's breed and age. Regular activity is crucial for physical and mental well-being.

Weight Monitoring: Regularly monitor your dog's weight and adjust their diet and exercise routine accordingly.

12. Nutritional Supplements:

Individual Needs: Some dogs may benefit from nutritional supplements based on their age, breed, or specific health conditions. Consult your veterinarian before introducing supplements.

13. End-of-Life Care and Decision-Making:

Quality of Life Discussions: When your dog reaches the senior stage, your veterinarian can help guide discussions about end-of-life care, pain management, and the decision-making process.

Compassionate Support: Veterinarians provide compassionate support during challenging times, offering guidance on euthanasia and aftercare options.

14. Microchipping and Identification:

Microchip Implantation: Ensure your dog is microchipped for identification in case they get lost. Keep contact information updated with the microchip registry.

15. Regular Grooming and Skin Care:

Skin Checks: Regularly check your dog's skin for signs of allergies, infections, or parasites. Seek veterinary advice if you notice any abnormalities.

Grooming Recommendations: Depending on your dog's breed, regular grooming may be necessary to maintain their coat and skin health.

Introducing New Foods Gradually

7.1 The Importance of Gradual Transitions

Making changes to your dog's diet, routine, or environment requires thoughtful consideration, especially when it comes to implementing gradual transitions. Whether it's a shift in their food, living arrangements, or daily schedule, introducing adjustments slowly is key to ensuring your dog's comfort, health, and overall well-being. Here's a look at why gradual transitions are crucial for your canine companion:

1. Digestive Sensitivity:
Gentle Adaptation: Dogs can have sensitive stomachs, and abrupt changes to their diet can lead to digestive upset. Gradual transitions allow their digestive system to adapt slowly to new foods without causing stress or discomfort.

Reduced Risk of Upset Stomach: Transitioning over a period of 7 to 10 days by mixing old and new food in increasing proportions minimizes the risk of diarrhea, vomiting, or other gastrointestinal issues.

2. Preventing Behavioral Stress:

Routine Comfort: Dogs thrive on routine and familiarity. Sudden changes can cause stress and anxiety, leading to behavioral issues. Gradual transitions provide a sense of continuity and comfort.

Positive Association: Whether it's a new living space or a modified daily routine, introducing changes slowly helps your dog build positive associations and adapt at their own pace.

3. Maintaining Emotional Well-Being:

Emotional Stability: Dogs form strong bonds with their owners and their environment. Abrupt changes, such as relocations or major lifestyle shifts, can impact their emotional stability. Gradual transitions offer a smoother adjustment process.

Supporting Confidence: Dogs build confidence when faced with changes at a pace they can handle. Gradual transitions allow them to explore and adapt while feeling secure.

4. Adapting to New Environments:

Familiarization: Moving to a new home or introducing a new pet requires time for familiarization. Gradual transitions allow your dog to explore and become comfortable with their new surroundings.

Minimizing Stressors: Reducing the speed of change minimizes potential stressors associated with new environments, helping your dog feel more at ease.

5. Dietary Changes and Nutrient Adaptation:

Avoiding Dietary Upsets: When switching dog food brands or formulations, gradual transitions help your dog adjust to new flavors and nutrient profiles. It also allows the digestive system to adapt to different ingredient compositions.

Balanced Nutrition: Over time, gradual transitions ensure that your dog receives a balanced and complete nutritional intake, avoiding sudden shifts that may impact their overall health.

6. Training and Behavior Modification:

Step-by-Step Training: Introducing new commands, behaviors, or training techniques gradually helps your dog understand and respond positively. Incremental changes provide them with the opportunity to learn at a comfortable pace.

Positive Reinforcement: Positive reinforcement during training is more effective when applied gradually. It allows your dog to associate new behaviors with positive experiences.

7. Medical Considerations:

Medication and Supplements: When introducing new medications or supplements, a gradual approach can help monitor your dog's response and minimize the risk of adverse reactions.

Veterinary Guidance: Always follow veterinary recommendations for transitioning to new medications or treatments, ensuring your dog's health and safety.

8. Weight Management:

Dietary Adjustments: If you're modifying your dog's diet for weight management, gradual transitions help control calorie intake and prevent sudden changes in weight that can impact their health.

Lifestyle Changes: Adjustments to exercise routines should also be gradual, especially for dogs transitioning from a sedentary lifestyle to a more active one.

9. Preventing Allergies and Sensitivities:

Identifying Triggers: Gradual transitions help identify potential allergies or sensitivities by allowing you to monitor your dog's response to new foods, environments, or products.

Timely Adjustments: If allergies or sensitivities arise, gradual transitions make it easier to pinpoint the cause and make timely adjustments to prevent prolonged discomfort.

10. Building Trust and Bond:

Trust-Building Process: Consistent, gradual changes build trust between you and your dog. It reinforces the bond by demonstrating that you are attuned to their needs and respect their individual pace.

Positive Interaction: Whether it's introducing a new family member, pet, or caregiver, gradual transitions ensure positive interactions, fostering a harmonious environment.

7.2 Monitoring for Allergic Reactions

While dogs can develop allergies to various substances, it's essential for pet owners to be vigilant and proactive in monitoring for potential allergic reactions. Allergic responses can manifest in various ways, affecting the skin, digestive system, or respiratory system. Here's a comprehensive guide on how to monitor your dog for allergic reactions and take prompt action when needed:

1. Understanding Common Allergens:

Food Allergies: Ingredients such as certain proteins, grains, or additives in dog food can trigger allergic reactions.

Environmental Allergens: Pollens, molds, dust mites, and certain plants can cause allergies in dogs.

Contact Allergens: Some dogs may develop skin reactions to certain fabrics, cleaning products, or grooming items.

2. Common Signs of Allergic Reactions:

Skin Issues: Itching, redness, hives, or hot spots on the skin are common signs of allergic reactions.

Digestive Upset: Vomiting, diarrhea, or changes in bowel habits may indicate a food allergy.

Respiratory Symptoms: Sneezing, coughing, or wheezing can occur in response to environmental allergens.

Ear Infections: Allergies can contribute to recurrent ear infections, with symptoms like head shaking, scratching, or foul odor.

3. Monitoring Changes in Behavior:

Lethargy: Allergic reactions may cause fatigue or a decrease in overall energy levels.

Changes in Appetite: Loss of appetite or increased thirst may be indicative of underlying allergies.

Restlessness or Agitation: Behavioral changes, such as restlessness or irritability, can signal discomfort.

4. Skin and Coat Observations:

Scratching and Biting: Persistent scratching, licking, or biting at certain body parts may indicate skin irritation.

Redness or Inflammation: Check for redness, inflammation, or rashes on the skin, especially around the paws, face, ears, and belly.

5. Digestive System Monitoring:

Vomiting and Diarrhea: Frequent vomiting or diarrhea can be signs of allergic reactions to food or environmental factors.

Changes in Stool: Monitor for changes in the color, consistency, or frequency of your dog's stool.

6. Respiratory System Observations:

Coughing or Sneezing: Allergies may manifest as respiratory symptoms, including coughing or sneezing.

Labored Breathing: If your dog shows signs of difficulty breathing, seek immediate veterinary attention.

7. Ear and Eye Checks:

Redness or Discharge: Red, inflamed eyes or abnormal discharge can be symptoms of allergies.

Ear Scratching or Odor: Frequent ear scratching, head shaking, or a foul odor from the ears may indicate allergic reactions.

8. Prompt Veterinary Attention:

Consultation with Veterinarian: If you suspect your dog is experiencing an allergic reaction, consult your veterinarian promptly. They can conduct allergy testing, recommend treatment options, and provide guidance on managing allergies.

Emergency Care: In severe cases, such as difficulty breathing or anaphylactic reactions, seek emergency veterinary care immediately.

9. Elimination Diets for Food Allergies:

Consultation with Veterinarian: If food allergies are suspected, your veterinarian may recommend an elimination diet to identify the specific allergen.

Strict Compliance: Follow the elimination diet guidelines provided by your veterinarian diligently to achieve accurate results.

10. Environmental Modifications:

Allergen Reduction: Take steps to reduce exposure to environmental allergens. This may include using air purifiers, keeping living spaces clean, and avoiding certain outdoor areas during peak allergy seasons.

11. Allergy Testing:

Skin or Blood Tests: Allergy testing conducted by a veterinarian can help identify specific allergens triggering your dog's reactions.

Customized Treatment Plans: Based on the results, your veterinarian can create a customized treatment plan, which may include medications, immunotherapy, or dietary changes.

12. Preventive Measures:

Regular Veterinary Check-ups: Schedule regular check-ups with your veterinarian to monitor your dog's overall health and address potential allergy concerns proactively.

Hygienic Practices: Keep your dog's living space clean, groom them regularly, and use pet-friendly cleaning products to minimize exposure to potential allergens.

13. Avoiding Triggers:

Identifying and Eliminating: Once specific triggers are identified, work with your veterinarian to develop strategies to avoid or minimize exposure to those allergens.

Educating Pet Care Providers: Inform pet care providers, such as groomers or boarding facilities, about your dog's allergies and specific needs.

7.3 Consulting with Your Veterinarian

Effective communication with your veterinarian is a cornerstone of responsible pet ownership, ensuring the well-being and longevity of your furry companion. Whether you're seeking preventive care, addressing health concerns, or navigating lifestyle changes, open and regular consultations with your veterinarian are essential. Here's a comprehensive guide on the importance of consulting with your veterinarian and how it contributes to your pet's overall health:

1. Routine Wellness Examinations:

Scheduled Check-ups: Regular wellness examinations, typically once a year for adult dogs and more frequently for puppies, seniors, or those with specific health concerns, are essential for preventive care.

Comprehensive Assessments: These exams involve thorough physical examinations, dental evaluations, and discussions about diet, behavior, and lifestyle.

2. Vaccinations and Preventive Care:

Customized Vaccination Plans: Veterinarians tailor vaccination plans based on your dog's age, breed, lifestyle, and risk factors.

Parasite Prevention: Regular preventive measures for parasites, including fleas, ticks, heartworms, and intestinal worms, are discussed and implemented.

3. Nutritional Guidance:

Dietary Recommendations: Veterinarians provide guidance on selecting the right commercial dog food or assist in creating a balanced homemade diet.

Weight Management: Recommendations for portion control, feeding schedules, and weight monitoring contribute to maintaining a healthy weight.

4. Dental Care:

Importance of Dental Health: Dental issues can impact overall health. Veterinarians may recommend dental cleanings, dental diets, or at-home dental care routines.

Regular Dental Check-ups: Periodic dental check-ups help identify and address dental problems early on.

5. Behavioral Consultations:

Understanding Behavior Changes: If you notice changes in your dog's behavior, your veterinarian can assess whether there are underlying health issues or behavioral concerns.

Training and Socialization Guidance: Veterinarians offer advice on training, socialization, and addressing behavioral challenges.

6. Senior Dog Care:

Increased Frequency of Check-ups: Senior dogs often require more frequent veterinary visits. Regular screenings for conditions like arthritis, kidney disease, and cognitive decline become essential.

Adjustments for Aging: Dietary changes, exercise recommendations, and preventive measures are tailored to address the unique needs of senior dogs.

7. Diagnostic Testing:

Proactive Health Monitoring: Blood work, urinalysis, and imaging studies are conducted to identify and monitor health conditions such as kidney disease, diabetes, or organ dysfunction.

Early Detection: Regular diagnostic testing allows for the early detection and management of potential health issues.

8. Spaying and Neutering:

Timing and Considerations: Veterinarians provide guidance on the optimal timing for spaying or neutering based on factors such as breed, size, and overall health.

9. Emergency Preparedness:

Emergency Contact Information: Veterinarians provide emergency contact information. Knowing where to seek emergency veterinary care is crucial in unforeseen situations.

First Aid Guidance: Veterinarians may offer advice on assembling a basic first aid kit for your dog and provide guidance on responding to common emergencies.

10. Ongoing Communication:

Open Dialogue: Regular communication with your veterinarian fosters a partnership in your dog's care. Discuss any concerns, changes in behavior, or potential health issues promptly.

Follow-Up Visits: Follow-up visits after treatments or surgeries allow your veterinarian to monitor your dog's recovery and adjust care as needed.

11. Weight and Exercise Management:

Guidance for Exercise: Veterinarians provide recommendations for appropriate exercise based on your dog's breed, age, and health status.

Regular Weight Monitoring: Monitoring your dog's weight and adjusting their diet and exercise routine as needed contributes to maintaining a healthy weight.

12. Nutritional Supplements:

Individualized Advice: Veterinarians can offer guidance on the need for nutritional supplements based on your dog's age, breed, or specific health conditions.

Quality and Dosage Recommendations: They provide information on choosing high-quality supplements and ensuring appropriate dosages.

13. End-of-Life Care and Decision-Making:

Quality of Life Discussions: In the senior stages, veterinarians help guide discussions about end-of-life care, pain management, and the decision-making process.

Compassionate Support: Veterinarians provide compassionate support during challenging times, offering guidance on euthanasia and aftercare options.

14. Microchipping and Identification:

Microchip Implantation: Veterinarians may recommend microchipping for identification in case your dog gets lost. Keeping contact information updated is crucial.

15. Regular Grooming and Skin Care:

Skin Checks: Regularly checking your dog's skin for signs of allergies, infections, or parasites is crucial. Veterinarians can provide guidance on skin care and grooming.

Consulting with your veterinarian is not only about addressing health issues but also about preventive care, fostering a trusting relationship, and ensuring a high quality of life for your dog. By actively engaging with your veterinarian, you contribute to the overall health, happiness, and longevity of your beloved canine companion.

Common Pitfalls and Challenges

8.1 Identifying and Avoiding High-Fat Traps

Maintaining a balanced and nutritious diet is crucial for your dog's well-being, and part of this involves being mindful of the fat content in their food. While some fats are essential for your dog's health, excessive intake can lead to obesity and related health issues. Here's a comprehensive guide on identifying and avoiding high-fat traps in your dog's diet:

1. Understanding Dietary Fats:

Essential Fats: Fats play a vital role in your dog's diet, providing energy, supporting skin and coat health, and aiding nutrient absorption.

Healthy Sources: Focus on incorporating healthy fats from sources like fish oil, flaxseed, and chicken fat into your dog's diet.

2. Identifying High-Fat Traps:

Commercial Treats: Many commercial dog treats, especially those labeled as high-value or with added flavor, can be high in fats. Check the nutritional information on packaging.

Table Scraps: Sharing human food, especially fatty leftovers or greasy items, can contribute to an excessive fat intake for your dog.

Certain Dog Foods: Some dog foods, particularly those designed for specific health conditions or life stages, may have higher fat content. Always check the labels.

Human Food Hazards: Foods like bacon, sausages, and fried items are not only high in fat but may also contain ingredients harmful to dogs.

3. Reading Dog Food Labels:

Focus on Percentage: Check the percentage of fat in the guaranteed analysis section of the dog food label. This indicates the proportion of fat by weight.

Differentiate Between Types of Fat: Understand the breakdown of fats into categories like saturated, unsaturated, and omega-3 fatty acids.

4. Balancing Fat Intake:

Consider Individual Needs: Dogs have varying energy requirements based on factors such as breed, age, activity level, and health status. Consult with your veterinarian to determine the appropriate fat levels for your dog.

Weight Management: Adjust fat intake to maintain a healthy weight for your dog. Overfeeding fats can contribute to obesity, leading to various health issues.

5. Health Risks of High-Fat Diets:

Obesity: Excessive fat consumption is a leading cause of obesity in dogs. Obesity contributes to various health problems, including joint issues, diabetes, and cardiovascular issues.

Pancreatitis: A sudden intake of high-fat foods can trigger pancreatitis, a painful and potentially serious inflammation of the pancreas.

Digestive Upset: High-fat diets can lead to digestive issues such as diarrhea, vomiting, and abdominal discomfort.

6. Selecting Low-Fat Treats:

Homemade Treats: Consider preparing homemade treats using lean protein sources and healthy fats. This allows you to control the ingredients and fat content.

Commercial Options: Look for commercially available low-fat treats with clear nutritional information. Choose treats designed for your dog's size and breed.

7. Balancing Omega-3 and Omega-6 Fatty Acids:

Importance of Balance: Both omega-3 and omega-6 fatty acids are essential for your dog's health. Ensure a balanced ratio between these two types of fats in their diet.

Sources of Omega-3s: Include sources like fish oil, flaxseed, and chia seeds for a healthy omega-3 intake.

8. Consulting with Your Veterinarian:

Individualized Guidance: Your veterinarian can provide tailored advice on your dog's dietary needs, considering factors like age, breed, health conditions, and activity level.

Monitoring Health: Regular veterinary check-ups help monitor your dog's weight, nutritional status, and overall health, allowing for timely adjustments to their diet.

9. Gradual Diet Changes:

Avoid Sudden Shifts: When transitioning to a new diet, whether it's a different dog food or homemade meals, do so gradually. This helps your dog's digestive system adjust and reduces the risk of gastrointestinal upset.

8.2 Dealing with Picky Eaters

Encountering a picky eater in your canine companion can be a challenge, but with patience, creativity, and a strategic approach, you can encourage healthier eating habits. Picky eating in dogs may stem from various reasons, including taste preferences, health issues, or behavioral factors. Here's a comprehensive guide on dealing with picky eaters and promoting a well-balanced diet:

1. Understand the Root Cause:

Health Considerations: Rule out any underlying health issues by consulting with your veterinarian. Dental problems, gastrointestinal discomfort, or other health concerns can contribute to picky eating.

Behavioral Factors: Some dogs may develop picky eating habits due to stress, changes in routine, or a dislike for specific textures or flavors.

2. Establish a Consistent Feeding Routine:

Scheduled Meals: Establish a regular feeding schedule to create a sense of routine and predictability.

Limited Time for Meals: Offer meals for a set duration (usually 15-20 minutes) and then remove the food bowl. This encourages dogs to eat within a specific timeframe.

3. Choose High-Quality, Palatable Food:

Varied Flavors and Textures: Experiment with different flavors and textures to identify what your dog prefers. Some dogs may prefer kibble, while others may enjoy wet or raw food.

High-Quality Ingredients: Opt for high-quality dog food with nutritious ingredients to enhance the palatability of the meal.

4. Avoid Overuse of Treats:

Limit Treats: If your dog is often given treats between meals, they may be less motivated to eat their regular meals. Limit treat intake to encourage a healthy appetite for regular food.

Use Treats Strategically: Use treats as rewards for finishing meals rather than offering them freely throughout the day.

5. Warm Up or Enhance the Food:

Temperature Matters: Some dogs prefer their food slightly warmed. Experiment with serving food at room temperature or warming it up slightly.

Add Toppers: Sprinkle small amounts of dog-friendly toppers, such as broth, plain yogurt, or bits of lean meat, to make the meal more enticing.

6. Be Mindful of Portion Sizes:

Appropriate Portions: Avoid overfeeding. Offer appropriate portion sizes to prevent obesity while ensuring your dog gets the necessary nutrients.

Consult with Veterinarian: Consult with your veterinarian to determine the appropriate portion size based on your dog's size, age, and activity level.

7. Limit Access to Table Scraps:

Discourage Begging: Avoid feeding your dog directly from the table or sharing human food, as this can contribute to picky eating behaviors.

Consistent Rules: Establish consistent rules for feeding to avoid confusion and reinforce good behavior.

8. Rotate Dog Food Brands or Flavors:

Change in Rotation: Rotate between different brands or flavors of dog food to provide variety and prevent boredom with a particular type of food.

Gradual Transition: Introduce changes gradually to avoid digestive upset.

9. Create a Positive Feeding Environment:

Quiet and Calm Setting: Ensure a calm and quiet environment during meals. Dogs may be less likely to eat if there are distractions or stressors.

Positive Reinforcement: Offer praise and positive reinforcement when your dog eats their meals, reinforcing the idea that mealtime is a positive experience.

10. Consult with a Professional Trainer:

Behavioral Modification: If picky eating is linked to behavioral issues, consider consulting with a professional dog trainer to address underlying concerns.

Positive Reinforcement Training: Positive reinforcement training can be effective in encouraging positive behaviors, including eating.

11. Monitor Weight and Overall Health:

Regular Vet Check-ups: Schedule regular veterinary check-ups to monitor your dog's weight and overall health. Address any concerns about picky eating during these visits.

Nutritional Supplements: Consult with your veterinarian to determine if nutritional supplements are necessary to ensure your dog receives essential nutrients.

12. Homemade Dog Treats or Meals:

DIY Options: Experiment with homemade treats or meals using dog-friendly ingredients. Ensure the recipes are nutritionally balanced and consult with your veterinarian for guidance.

13. Patience and Consistency:

Gradual Changes: Make changes to your dog's diet gradually to allow them to adjust.

Consistent Approach: Be consistent in your approach to feeding, creating a routine that your dog can rely on.

14. Seek Veterinary Advice for Persistent Issues:

Professional Guidance: If your dog's picky eating persists or is accompanied by weight loss or health concerns, seek professional veterinary advice promptly.

Underlying Health Issues: Your veterinarian can conduct tests to rule out underlying health issues and provide tailored recommendations for your dog's unique needs.

8.3 Addressing Digestive Issues

Maintaining a healthy digestive system is essential for your dog's overall well-being. Digestive issues can manifest in various forms, including diarrhea, vomiting, constipation, or signs of discomfort. Addressing these concerns requires a combination of understanding potential causes, implementing preventive measures, and seeking veterinary guidance. Here's a comprehensive guide to help you navigate and address digestive issues in your canine companion:

1. Recognizing Common Signs of Digestive Issues:

Diarrhea: Loose, watery stools can indicate digestive upset.

Vomiting: Occasional vomiting may be normal, but persistent or severe vomiting requires attention.

Constipation: Difficulty in passing stools or infrequent bowel movements may signal digestive issues.

Changes in Appetite: A sudden loss of appetite or excessive hunger can be indicative of digestive problems.

Flatulence and Discomfort: Frequent gas, abdominal pain, or signs of discomfort during and after meals may suggest digestive concerns.

2. Assessing Potential Causes:

Dietary Changes: Abrupt changes in diet or introduction of new foods can lead to digestive upset. Gradual transitions are crucial.

Food Allergies or Intolerances: Allergies or sensitivities to certain ingredients in the diet can contribute to digestive issues.

Parasitic Infections: Internal parasites, such as worms, can cause gastrointestinal problems.

Bacterial or Viral Infections: Infections from bacteria or viruses can lead to diarrhea and other digestive symptoms.

Ingestion of Foreign Objects: Dogs may ingest items that can obstruct the digestive tract, leading to issues.

Pancreatitis: Inflammation of the pancreas can cause digestive problems, especially if your dog consumes high-fat foods.

3. Immediate Actions for Mild Digestive Upset:

Temporary Fasting: Withhold food for 12-24 hours to allow the digestive system to rest. Provide access to water to prevent dehydration.

Bland Diet: Gradually reintroduce a bland diet, such as boiled chicken and rice, to soothe the digestive tract.

Probiotics: Consider adding canine-specific probiotics to promote a healthy balance of gut bacteria.

4. Gradual Food Transitions:

Introduce Changes Slowly: When switching dog food or making dietary changes, do so gradually over 7-10 days to prevent digestive upset.

Monitor Responses: Observe your dog's response to new foods, noting any signs of discomfort, diarrhea, or vomiting.

5. Consult with Your Veterinarian:

Persistent Symptoms: If digestive issues persist or worsen, consult your veterinarian promptly.

Diagnostic Tests: Your vet may recommend tests, such as fecal exams, bloodwork, or imaging, to identify the underlying cause.

6. Dietary Considerations:

Prescription Diets: In some cases, veterinarians may recommend prescription diets designed for digestive health.

Novel Protein Diets: For dogs with suspected food allergies, novel protein diets may be advised to identify and eliminate triggers.

7. Hydration and Electrolyte Balance:

Prevent Dehydration: Ensure your dog has access to clean, fresh water at all times to prevent dehydration.

Electrolyte Replenishment: In cases of severe diarrhea or vomiting, your veterinarian may recommend electrolyte solutions to restore balance.

8. Parasite Prevention and Treatment:

Regular Deworming: Follow a deworming schedule as recommended by your veterinarian to prevent and address internal parasites.

Flea and Tick Control: Parasites like fleas can transmit intestinal parasites. Use preventive measures.

9. Avoiding Harmful Substances:

Toxic Foods: Keep dogs away from foods toxic to them, such as chocolate, onions, garlic, and certain artificial sweeteners.

Household Hazards: Ensure your dog cannot access household items, plants, or chemicals that may be harmful if ingested.

10. Pancreatitis Management:

Low-Fat Diets: If pancreatitis is a concern, your veterinarian may recommend a low-fat diet.

Medication: Medications to manage inflammation or pain may be prescribed.

11. Monitoring and Follow-Up:

Observing Stool Quality: Monitor the quality of your dog's stools. Consistency, color, and any signs of blood are important indicators.

Regular Vet Check-ups: Schedule regular veterinary check-ups, especially for senior dogs or those with chronic digestive issues.

12. Lifestyle and Stress Management:

Consistent Routine: Dogs thrive on routine. Maintain a consistent feeding schedule and daily routine.

Minimize Stressors: Identify and minimize sources of stress, as stress can contribute to digestive issues.

13. Long-Term Dietary Planning:

Tailored Nutrition: Work with your veterinarian to determine the most appropriate long-term diet based on your dog's age, breed, health status, and any dietary restrictions.

14. Educating Care Providers:

Informing Groomers and Boarding Facilities: Provide information about your dog's digestive sensitivities to groomers or boarding facilities to ensure appropriate care.

Addressing digestive issues requires a holistic approach, considering both immediate actions and long-term management. Regular communication with your veterinarian, a focus on preventive care, and a watchful eye on your dog's overall health are key components of ensuring a healthy digestive system for your canine companion.

CONCLUSION

9.1 Looking Ahead to a Healthy Future for Your Dog

Ensuring a healthy and vibrant future for your dog involves a commitment to proactive care, preventive measures, and an understanding of their evolving needs. As your loyal companion ages, thoughtful planning and attention to various aspects of their well-being become paramount. Here's a comprehensive guide to help you look ahead to a healthy future for your beloved canine:

1. Keeping up with Customary Veterinary Check-ups:
Scheduled Wellness Examinations: Regular veterinary check-ups, typically annually or as recommended by your veterinarian, are crucial for preventive care.
Early Detection: Routine screenings can help detect potential health issues early, allowing for timely intervention.
2. Tailoring Nutrition to Your Dog's Life Stage:
Age-Appropriate Diets: As your dog ages, their nutritional needs may change. Transition to age-appropriate diets to address evolving requirements.

Specialized Diets: Certain health conditions or breeds may benefit from specialized diets. Consult your veterinarian for personalized recommendations.

3. Weight Management for Longevity:

Maintaining a Healthy Weight: Obesity can contribute to various health issues. Monitor your dog's weight and adjust diet and exercise accordingly.

Consult with Veterinarian: Seek guidance from your veterinarian on an optimal weight management plan based on your dog's age, breed, and activity level.

4. Caring for Dental Health:

Regular Dental Check-ups: Dental issues can impact overall health. Schedule regular dental check-ups and cleanings to prevent periodontal disease.

At-Home Dental Care: Implement an at-home dental care routine, such as tooth brushing or dental chews, to promote oral health.

5. Ensuring Adequate Exercise and Mental Stimulation:

Adapting Exercise Routine: Adjust the intensity and duration of exercise as your dog ages. Regular activity is crucial for physical and mental well-being.

Mental Stimulation: Engage your dog with interactive toys, puzzles, and new experiences to keep their mind active and prevent boredom.

6. Monitoring Joint Health:

Supplementation: Consider joint supplements, especially for breeds prone to joint issues or senior dogs. Talk about choices with your veterinarian.

Low-Impact Exercise: Opt for low-impact exercises, such as swimming or gentle walks, to support joint health.

7. Forestalling and Overseeing Constant Circumstances:

Regular Health Screenings: Screen for common age-related conditions, such as arthritis, diabetes, or kidney disease, through regular veterinary visits.

Medication Adherence: If your dog requires medication for chronic conditions, ensure consistent adherence to prescribed treatment plans.

8. Grooming and Skin Care:

Regular Inspection: Conduct regular skin checks for lumps, bumps, or changes in coat quality. Report any worries to your veterinarian.

Gentle Grooming: As dogs age, they may require gentler grooming practices. Use soft brushes and be mindful of any discomfort.

9. Eye and Ear Care:

Routine Eye Exams: Regular eye exams can detect conditions like cataracts or glaucoma early on. Talk about with your veterinarian.

Ear Cleaning: Keep ears clean and dry to prevent infections, especially in breeds prone to ear issues.

10. Quality Sleep and Comfort:

Comfortable Bedding: Provide a comfortable and supportive bed, especially for senior dogs with arthritis or joint pain.

Environmental Considerations: Ensure a quiet and comfortable environment for quality sleep, essential for overall well-being.

11. Maintaining Emotional Well-being:

Quality Time: Spend quality time with your dog through play, walks, and cuddles. Dogs thrive on companionship.

Recognizing Behavioral Changes: Be attentive to behavioral changes, as they may indicate discomfort or underlying health issues.

12. Age-Appropriate Vaccinations:

Consult with Veterinarian: Work with your veterinarian to determine the necessary vaccinations based on your dog's age, lifestyle, and health status.

Booster Shots: Keep vaccinations up to date with booster shots as recommended by your veterinarian.

13. Emergency Preparedness:

Emergency Kit: Prepare a pet emergency kit with essential supplies, including medical records, medications, and contact information for your veterinarian.

Emergency Plan: Have a plan in place for evacuation or seeking emergency veterinary care in unforeseen situations.

14. Creating a Will and Estate Plan:

Pet Provisions: Include provisions for your dog in your will or estate plan, specifying a trusted caregiver and detailing your pet's needs.

Communication with Caretakers: Share important information about your dog's health, preferences, and routines with designated caretakers.

15. Embracing Senior-Specific Care:

Geriatric Health Monitoring: For senior dogs, consider more frequent veterinary check-ups and geriatric health screenings.

Comfort Measures: Implement additional comfort measures, such as heated beds for arthritis relief or softer food for dental comfort.

16. End-of-Life Arranging with Empathy:

Quality of Life Assessments: Regularly assess your dog's quality of life, considering factors like pain, mobility, and overall happiness.

Compassionate End-of-Life Decisions: If necessary, consult with your veterinarian about end-of-life decisions, ensuring your dog's comfort and dignity.

17. Continual Learning and Adaptation:

Stay Informed: Keep abreast of developments in veterinary care and nutritional science to adapt your dog's care plan as needed.

Consultation with Veterinarian: Regularly consult with your veterinarian for guidance on evolving care requirements.

Looking ahead to a healthy future for your dog involves a thoughtful combination of proactive health measures, compassionate care, and a commitment to adapting their lifestyle as they age. By fostering a strong partnership with your veterinarian and addressing evolving needs, you can provide your canine companion with a fulfilling and vibrant life throughout their golden years.

www.ingramcontent.com/pod-product-compliance
Lightning Source LLC
Chambersburg PA
CBHW071051290526
45795CB00004B/1436